The Unique Path

Life Crisis Management

BY

Dr. Troy Foskey Jr

RAVEN-WOLF MEDIA, LLP
2018

DEDICATION

I dedicate this, my first book to those who matter most in my life & to those who said I'd never accomplish anything. These two sides of the same coin have contributed to my drive, my ambition, my ability to accomplish my goals regardless of the obstacles.

Thank you to the ones that stuck it out when it might have been easier to run. Thank you **Melissa, Pepa, Mema, Danny, & Jamie.** I love you all. Each one of you have loved me, and supported my dreams, and have been by my side through the very worst of times. I am humbled, & grateful beyond words!

Thank you & I love you to my Children, ***Shayne Ireland Foskey* & *Alex Andrew Crays*.** You can conquer the world, or be crushed by its weight. Only you can choose which path you journey down. So, Suck it Up & drive on! Choose Your Own Unique Path To Greatness!

A warm & sincere heartfelt Thank You to my dear friends, who are just like family & in many ways, better. My Friend & Director of Patient Relations, **Heather Jo Rhymes, LPT, EMT-A & Michael Alex Adkins,** you have both been there when it counts & you have my unending appreciation & loyalty.

Thank you to the US Air Force & the US Army, both taught me how to survive the not so survivable & to shoot for my target...and hit it!...Everytime! Hooah!

A Special Thank you to the late **Sheriff Cecil Nobles of Long County GA.** He knew what second chances meant & when to give them.

And to those who said that I'd never accomplish anything. . . You know who you are. . . I thank you for being better than any Drill Instructor or Alarm Clock! I woke up each day & I overcame the barriers to my Own *Unique Path* & your voices lit my way!

INTRODUCTION

This is the first book in a series that will outline & detail ways to treat and manage Life Crisis Issues/disorders such as PTSD, Suicide, Bullying, Anxiety, Sexual Assault, Relationship Problems, Depression, Social Anxiety, Eating Disorders, & many more.

The Unique Path series will begin with this, my First book,

THE UNIQUE PATH: LIFE CRISIS MANAGEMENT

The Unique Path System is a new system of treatment for Life Crisis & other issues based upon Humanistic & Holistic Principles, Self Discipline, Fundamental Medicine, & a LifeTime of experience & training. This new system of treatment is being developed by

Dr. Troy Foskey Jr.
The Raven Institute, Inc.
All rights reserved.

In this first book of The Unique Path series, I will discuss and detail common Life Crisis Issues and the ways that they're typically treated & managed. Please note that in this, the first book, I'm focusing on information that is generally known as "Traditional", or "The Norm". I am not providing treatment, management, or coaching methods for these disorders using the techniques I created in **The Unique Path** system. This book provides information & "traditional" professional treatment advice/methods for each of the major Life Crisis issues & disorders discussed in this first installment. I will be publishing additional books very soon, July 2018, detailing methods of dealing with these issues & disorders, as well as many more topics, using **The Unique Path** system. This book is an introduction and its purpose is to familiarize readers with these Life Crisis issues & disorders.

I want to extend my sincere, & humble thanks to you all for reading my book & I hope that you'll give each of my following books a try as well. I will always do my best to provide helpful, in depth, and universally useful information & treatment options, if applicable, about any issue/topic that I address. If anyone desires further information about any topic that I discuss, or wishes to seek help, treatment, or more in depth professional advice for their own Life Crisis issue, or that of a loved one, please contact me at:

Dr. Troy Foskey Jr

The Raven Institute, Inc. - Raven Crisis Care & Intervention

40 E Academy St Suite 826

Ludowici, GA 31316

www.facebook.com/ravencrisiscareintervention

Twitter: TroyFoskey_PhD

Take a look around me

Taking pages from a magazine

Been looking for the answer

Ever since we were seventeen

You know the truth can be a weapon

To fight this world of ill intentions

A new answer to the same question

How many times will you learn the same lesson?

I think they got it all wrong

We just got to hold on

And on, and on, and on

'Cause we're gonna be legends

Gonna get their attention

What we're doing here ain't just scary

It's about to be legendary

Yeah we're gonna be legends

Gonna teach 'em all a lesson

Got this feeling that we're so sweet caring

It's about to be legendary

- Wesley Arms
"LEGENDARY"

The Raven Institute, Inc.

CONTENTS

- PTSD
- HRV
- ANXIETY
- SUICIDE PREVENTION
- DEPRESSION
- ADHD
- SUBSTANCE ABUSE
- OCD
- SOCIAL ANXIETY
- EATING DISORDERS
- ABOUT THE AUTHOR

1

Post-Traumatic Stress Disorder

PTSD is a disorder that develops in some people who have experienced a shocking, scary, or dangerous event.

It is natural to feel afraid during and after a traumatic situation. Fear triggers many split-second changes in the body to help defend against danger or to avoid it. This "fight-or-flight" response is a typical reaction meant to protect a person from harm. Nearly everyone will experience a range of reactions after trauma, yet most people recover from initial symptoms naturally. Those who continue to experience problems may be diagnosed with PTSD. People who have PTSD may feel stressed or frightened even when they are not in danger.

Not every traumatized person develops ongoing (chronic) or even short-term (acute) PTSD. Not everyone with PTSD has been through a dangerous event. Some experiences, like the sudden, unexpected death of a loved one, can also cause PTSD. Symptoms usually begin early, within 3 months of the traumatic incident, but sometimes they begin years afterward. Symptoms must last more than a month and be severe enough to interfere with relationships or work to be considered PTSD. The course of the illness varies. Some people recover within 6 months, while others have symptoms that last much longer. In some people, the condition becomes chronic.

A doctor who has experience helping people with mental illnesses, such as a psychiatrist or psychologist, can diagnose PTSD.

To be diagnosed with PTSD, an adult must have all of the following for at least 1 month:

- At least one re-experiencing symptom
- At least one avoidance symptom
- At least two arousal and reactivity symptoms
- At least two cognition and mood symptoms

Re-experiencing symptoms include:

- Flashbacks—reliving the trauma over and over, including physical symptoms like a racing heart or sweating
- Bad dreams
- Frightening thoughts

Re-experiencing symptoms may cause problems in a person's everyday routine. The symptoms can start from the person's own thoughts and feelings. Words, objects, or situations that are reminders of the event can also trigger re-experiencing symptoms.

Avoidance symptoms include:

- Staying away from places, events, or objects that are reminders of the traumatic experience
- Avoiding thoughts or feelings related to the traumatic event

Things that remind a person of the traumatic event can trigger avoidance symptoms. These symptoms may cause a person to change his or her personal routine. For example, after a bad car accident, a person who usually drives may avoid driving or riding in a car.

Arousal and reactivity symptoms include:

- Being easily startled
- Feeling tense or "on edge"
- Having difficulty sleeping
- Having angry outbursts

Arousal symptoms are usually constant, instead of being triggered by things that remind one of the traumatic events. These symptoms can make the person feel stressed and angry. They may make it hard to do daily tasks, such as sleeping, eating, or concentrating.

Cognition and mood symptoms include:

- Trouble remembering key features of the traumatic event

- Negative thoughts about oneself or the world
- Distorted feelings like guilt or blame
- Loss of interest in enjoyable activities

Cognition and mood symptoms can begin or worsen after the traumatic event, but are not due to injury or substance use. These symptoms can make the person feel alienated or detached from friends or family members.

It is natural to have some of these symptoms after a dangerous event. Sometimes people have very serious symptoms that go away after a few weeks. This is called acute stress disorder, or ASD. When the symptoms last more than a month, seriously affect one's ability to function, and are not due to substance use, medical illness, or anything except the event itself, they might be PTSD. Some people with PTSD don't show any symptoms for weeks or months. PTSD is often accompanied by depression, substance abuse, or one or more of the other anxiety disorder.

Do Children React differently Than Adults?

Children and teens can have extreme reactions to trauma, but their symptoms may not be the same as adults. In very young children (less than 6 years of age), these symptoms can include:

- Wetting the bed after having learned to use the toilet
- Forgetting how to or being unable to talk
- Acting out the scary event during playtime
- Being unusually clingy with a parent or other adult

Older children and teens are more likely to show symptoms similar to those seen in adults. They may also develop disruptive, disrespectful, or destructive behaviors. Older children and teens may feel guilty for not preventing injury or deaths. They may also have thoughts of revenge.

Risk Factors

Anyone can develop PTSD at any age. This includes war veterans, children, and people who have been through a physical or sexual assault, abuse, accident, disaster, or many other serious events. According to the National Center for

PTSD, about 7 or 8 out of every 100 people will experience PTSD at some point in their lives. Women are more likely to develop PTSD than men, and genes may make some people more likely to develop PTSD than others.

Not everyone with PTSD has been through a dangerous event. Some people develop PTSD after a friend or family member experiences danger or harm. The sudden, unexpected death of a loved one can also lead to PTSD.

Why do some people develop PTSD and other people do not?

It is important to remember that not everyone who lives through a dangerous event develops PTSD. In fact, most people will not develop the disorder.

Many factors play a part in whether a person will develop PTSD. Some examples are listed below. *Risk factors* make a person more likely to develop PTSD. Other factors, called *resilience factors*, can help reduce the risk of the disorder.

Risk Factors and Resilience Factors for PTSD

Some factors that increase risk for PTSD include:

- Living through dangerous events and traumas
- Getting hurt
- Seeing another person hurt, or seeing a dead body
- Childhood trauma
- Feeling horror, helplessness, or extreme fear
- Having little or no social support after the event
- Dealing with extra stress after the event, such as loss of a loved one, pain and injury, or loss of a job or home
- Having a history of mental illness or substance abuse

Some resilience factors that may reduce the risk of PTSD Include:

- Seeking out support from other people, such as friends and family
- Finding a support group after a traumatic event
- Learning to feel good about one's own actions in the

face of danger

- Having a positive coping strategy, or a way of getting through the bad event and learning from it
- Being able to act and respond effectively despite feeling fear

Researchers are studying the importance of these and other risk and resilience factors, including genetics and neurobiology. With more research, someday it may be possible to predict who is likely to develop PTSD and to prevent it.

Treatments and Therapies

The main treatments for people with PTSD are medications, psychotherapy ("talk" therapy), or both. Everyone is different, and PTSD affects people differently so a treatment that works for one person may not work for another. It is important for anyone with PTSD to be treated by a mental health provider who is experienced with PTSD. Some people with PTSD need to try different treatments to find what works for their symptoms.

If someone with PTSD is going through an ongoing trauma, such as being in an abusive relationship, both of the problems need to be addressed. Other ongoing problems can include panic disorder, depression, substance abuse, and feeling suicidal.

Medications

The most studied medications for treating PTSD include antidepressants, which may help control PTSD symptoms such as sadness, worry, anger, and feeling numb inside. Antidepressants and other medications may be prescribed along with psychotherapy. Other medications may be helpful for specific PTSD symptoms. For example, although it is not currently FDA approved, research has shown that Prazosin may be helpful with sleep problems, particularly nightmares, commonly experienced by people with PTSD. Doctors and patients can work together to find the best medication or medication combination, as well as the right dose.

Psychotherapy

Psychotherapy (sometimes called "talk therapy") involves talking with a mental health professional to treat a mental illness. Psychotherapy can occur one-on-one or in a group. Talk therapy treatment for PTSD usually lasts 6 to 12 weeks, but it can last longer. Research shows that support from family and friends can be an important part of recovery.

Many types of psychotherapy can help people with PTSD. Some types target the symptoms of PTSD directly. Other therapies focus on social, family, or job-related problems. The doctor or therapist may combine different therapies depending on each person's needs.

Effective psychotherapies tend to emphasize a few key components, including education about symptoms, teaching skills to help identify the triggers of symptoms, and skills to manage the symptoms. One helpful form of therapy is called cognitive behavioral therapy, or CBT. CBT can include:

- Exposure therapy. This helps people face and control

their fear. It gradually exposes them to the trauma they experienced in a safe way. It uses imagining, writing, or visiting the place where the event happened. The therapist uses these tools to help people with PTSD cope with their feelings.

- Cognitive restructuring. This helps people make sense of the bad memories. Sometimes people remember the event differently than how it happened. They may feel guilt or shame about something that is not their fault. The therapist helps people with PTSD look at what happened in a realistic way.

There are other types of treatment that can help as well. People with PTSD should talk about all treatment options with a therapist. Treatment should equip individuals with the skills to manage their symptoms and help them participate in activities that they enjoyed before developing PTSD.

How Talk Therapies Help People Overcome PTSD

Talk therapies teach people helpful ways to react to the frightening events that trigger their PTSD symptoms. Based on this general goal, different types of therapy may:

- Teach about trauma and its effects
- Use relaxation and anger-control skills
- Provide tips for better sleep, diet, and exercise habits
- Help people identify and deal with guilt, shame, and other feelings about the event
- Focus on changing how people react to their PTSD symptoms.

For example, therapy helps people face reminders of the trauma.

Beyond Treatment: How can I help myself?

It may be very hard to take that first step to help yourself. It is important to realize that although it may take some time, with treatment, you can get better. If you are unsure where to go for help, ask your family doctor. You can also check NIMH's Help for Mental Illness Page or search online for "mental health providers," "social services," "hotlines," or "physicians" for phone numbers and addresses. An emergency room doctor can also provide temporary help and can tell you where and how to get further help.

To help yourself while in treatment:

- Talk with your doctor about treatment options
- Engage in mild physical activity or exercise to help reduce stress
- Set realistic goals for yourself
- Break up large tasks into small ones, set some priorities, and do what you can as you can
- Try to spend time with other people, and confide in a trusted friend or relative. Tell others about things that may trigger symptoms.
- Expect your symptoms to improve gradually, not immediately
- Identify and seek out comforting situations, places, and people

Caring for yourself and others is especially important when large numbers of people are exposed to traumatic events (such as natural disasters, accidents, and violent acts). For more information, see the Learn More section, below.

Next Steps for PTSD Research

In the last decade, progress in research on the mental and biological foundations of PTSD has lead scientists to focus on better understanding the underlying causes of why people experience a range of reactions to trauma.

- NIMH-funded researchers are exploring trauma patients in acute care settings to better understand the changes that occur in individuals whose symptoms improve naturally.
- Other research is looking at how fear memories are affected by learning, changes in the body, or even sleep.
- Research on preventing the development of PTSD soon after trauma exposure is also underway.
- Still other research is attempting to identify what factors determine whether someone with PTSD will respond well to one type of intervention or another, aiming to develop more personalized, effective, and

efficient treatments.

- As gene research and brain imaging technologies continue to improve, scientists are more likely to be able to pinpoint when and where in the brain PTSD begins. This understanding may then lead to better targeted treatments to suit each person's own needs or even prevent the disorder before it causes harm.

2
HEART RATE VARIABILITY

It isn't always the strongest or smartest who survive; often it's those who can adapt best to change. As one of life's Warriors, you probably know how important physical and mental adaptability is in order to navigate complex situations rapidly and efficiently. Did you know you can train your heart to be more responsive and efficient to meet those demands? One way your heart can help you do this is through heart rate variability, or HRV. Learn how to train your heart to help your body adapt quickly, effectively, and effortlessly to changing circumstances.

HRV is different from heart rate—the number of times your heart beats in a certain amount of time. HRV is a measure of how much time varies *between* heartbeats. HRV tells you not only how your heart is functioning but also how your brain is coping. When faced with a threat (real or imagined), your body initiates the fight or flight response, cueing your heart to pick up the pace and your breathing to quicken and shorten, which allows you to respond efficiently. Once your brain determines that the threat is gone, that response should turn off, allowing you to relax or return to your status quo.

Think of HRV like the responsiveness of a car. When you merge onto a freeway, you want your car to adjust quickly when you hit the gas and reach the desired speed as soon as possible after you hit the pedal. Then when it's time to slow down, you want a car that responds quickly when you hit the brakes, to bring you down to a safe speed. Think of the speed of the car as your heart rate and the ability to accelerate or decelerate quickly as your HRV. While heart rate alone can indicate how you're functioning, looking at heart rate and HRV together is a better indication of how you're managing stress and maintaining optimal levels of performance. Many cars can hit 60 mph, but only high-performance cars can move from 0 to 60 in 3.5 seconds.

Why does HRV matter?

Low HRV (less variation in time between heartbeats) is

linked to:

- fatigue during training
- negative mental health symptoms
- poorer physical health

Higher HRV (more variation in time between beats) is linked to optimized performance through:

- improved focus and attention
- better stress management
- better decision-making under pressure
- faster recovery from physical and psychological strain

The higher your HRV, the better your heart is able to adapt to changing demands.

Back to the example of a car's performance: Spending too much time in high gear causes wear and tear on your engine over time, so it's important to shift into a lower gear when the situation doesn't warrant being in high gear. And the more quickly you can downshift, the more you save energy and reduce the possibility of damage. On the other hand, being able to shift into high gear to deal quickly with a threat means you're able to stay more agile and ready to handle challenges. Higher HRV helps you shift gears quickly and effectively.

Training Your HRV

The good news is: You can train your HRV. If you have access to a biofeedback practitioner or cardiologist, you can seek the advice of a healthcare professional to get deeper insight into HRV. One way to train HRV on your own is through controlled breathing. Breathing in a rhythmic fashion can improve your HRV and strengthen your body's ability to shift between states of tension and relaxation.

Another training tool is progressive muscle relaxation or PMR, which can help improve mental health symptoms, reduce feelings of being keyed up or on edge, increase a sense of calm, and increase HRV by engaging the part of your nervous system that acts as your "brakes" for the fight or flight system. The goal of PMR is to bring awareness to how your body changes between states of stress and tension versus relaxation and calm. As you build this awareness over time, you become more able to notice when your body is stressed and you develop more control over that physical response.

3

ANXIETY

Most people equate feeling anxious or nervous with something bad, or it's a signal you're not prepared or mentally tough enough. But you can learn to embrace anxiety and use it to your advantage to improve your performance. Everyone has experienced the feeling of anxiety before—whether it's getting ready to head out on a new mission, bringing a child home from the hospital, or simply having to start a difficult conversation. It probably got in your way of being effective too.

In high-stakes situations where performance matters, the emotions and feelings in your body that go along with anxiety are common. Your heart beats faster, you might feel sweaty, and your stomach can feel uneasy. Even though these are signs your body is preparing you to be at your best, this nervousness can feel unpleasant, and your emotions and physical senses of anxiety often become a source of stress.

Take the example of having to give an important brief to a commander. As you're getting ready to speak, you might notice you're feeling anxious, and you might say to yourself, "I feel like this because I don't have my act together" or "I'm sweating because I can't handle this." Interpreting what's happening in your body as something negative then makes you even more likely to continue thinking negatively about yourself and your ability to manage the situation. And then that in turn reinforces your anxious feelings and fuels more of those uncomfortable physical sensations.

Why can't you just relax?

There are some strategies you can learn to help bring relief from stress. For example, Tactical Breathing can help you balance out your fight-or-flight stress response, calm down, and feel more in control. However, research shows there are times when trying to calm down can negatively impact your performance. When you're feeling anxious, it might be difficult—or even impossible—to simply "decide" to feel calmer mentally because it isn't consistent with what's happening in your body. And trying to pretend you're calm (when you know you aren't) can bring on even more anxiety.

Get Excited Instead!

How you interpret the physical sensations of anxiety can change how you feel emotionally—including your overall mindset—and ultimately make a difference in how you perform. When you're feeling really anxious, try instead to reinterpret your anxiety as excitement. Tell yourself the sensations you feel are signals your mind and body are preparing you to meet the challenge ahead, rather than a sign you can't handle what's going on.

It's normal to interpret some physical signs as performance anxiety. But because some of your body's reactions to excitement—increased heart rate, "butterflies," etc.—are the same as with anxiety, you actually can make the conscious choice to feel excited when you're anxious. This doesn't make your anxiety go away, but it enables you to feel more confident in the moment. Excitement feels good and puts your mind on a different track. When you're excited, it's also easier to view challenges as opportunities, not just potential threats.

Bottom Line

So when you feel anxious about performing on your Physical Fitness Test, speaking at a spouses' meeting, or helping your kid prepare for the big game, remember it's normal to feel anxious. Your Mindset About Stress and the anxiety in your life will determine whether the anxiety helps you perform your best or gets in your way. Excitement is anxiety's cousin: Convince yourself to feel excited, and in turn, enjoy a boost in performance.

4
Suicide Prevention

Suicide is a major public health concern. Over 40,000 people die by suicide each year in the United States; it is the 10th leading cause of death overall. Suicide is complicated and tragic but it is often preventable. Knowing the warning signs for suicide and how to get help can help save lives.

Signs and Symptoms

The behaviors listed below may be signs that someone is thinking about suicide.

- Talking about wanting to die or wanting to kill themselves
- Talking about feeling empty, hopeless, or having no reason to live
- Making a plan or looking for a way to kill themselves, such as searching online, stockpiling pills, or buying a

gun
- Talking about great guilt or shame
- Talking about feeling trapped or feeling that there are no solutions
- Feeling unbearable pain (emotional pain or physical pain)
- Talking about being a burden to others
- Using alcohol or drugs more often
- Acting anxious or agitated
- Withdrawing from family and friends
- Changing eating and/or sleeping habits
- Showing rage or talking about seeking revenge
- Taking great risks that could lead to death, such as driving extremely fast
- Talking or thinking about death often
- Displaying extreme mood swings, suddenly changing from very sad to very calm or happy
- Giving away important possessions
- Saying goodbye to friends and family
- Putting affairs in order, making a will

If these warning signs apply to you or someone you know, get help as soon as possible, particularly if the behavior is new or has increased recently. One resource is the National Suicide Prevention Lifeline, 1-800-273-TALK (8255). The Lifeline is available 24 hours a day, 7 days a week. The deaf and hard of hearing can contact the Lifeline via TTY at 1-800-799-4889.

Risk Factors

Suicide does not discriminate. People of all genders, ages, and ethnicities can be at risk. Suicidal behavior is complex and there is no single cause. In fact, many different factors contribute to someone making a suicide attempt. But people most at risk tend to share certain characteristics. The main risk factors for suicide are:

- Depression, other mental disorders, or substance abuse disorder

- Certain medical conditions
- Chronic pain
- A prior suicide attempt
- Family history of a mental disorder or substance abuse
- Family history of suicide
- Family violence, including physical or sexual abuse
- Having guns or other firearms in the home
- Having recently been released from prison or jail
- Being exposed to others' suicidal behavior, such as that of family members, peers, or celebrities

Many people have some of these risk factors but do not attempt suicide. It is important to note that suicide is not a normal response to stress. Suicidal thoughts or actions are a sign of extreme distress, not a harmless bid for attention, and should not be ignored.

Often, family and friends are the first to recognize the warning signs of suicide and can be the first step toward helping an at-risk individual find treatment with someone who specializes in diagnosing and treating mental health conditions.

Do gender and age affect suicide risk?

Men are more likely to die by suicide than women, but women are more likely to *attempt* suicide. Men are more likely to use deadlier methods, such as firearms or suffocation. Women are more likely than men to attempt suicide by poisoning. The most recent figures released by the CDC show that the highest rate of suicide deaths among women is found between ages 45 and 64, while the highest rate for men occurs at ages 75+. Children and young adults also are at risk for suicide. Suicide is the second leading cause of death for young people ages 15 to 34.

What about different racial/ethnic groups?

The CDC reports that among racial and ethnic groups, American Indians and Alaska Natives tend to have the highest rate of suicides, followed by non-Hispanic Whites. African Americans tend to have the lowest suicide rate, while Hispanics tend to have the second lowest rate.

5 Action Steps for Helping Someone in Emotional Pain

1. Ask: "Are you thinking about killing yourself?" It's not an easy question but studies show that asking at-risk individuals if they are suicidal does not increase suicides or suicidal thoughts.

2. Keep them safe: Reducing a suicidal person's access to highly lethal items or places is an important part of suicide prevention. While this is not always easy, asking if the at-risk person has a plan and removing or disabling the lethal meanscan make a difference.

3. Be there: Listen carefully and learn what the individual is thinking and feeling. Findings suggest acknowledging and talking about suicide may in fact reduce rather than increase suicidal thoughts.

4. Help them connect: Save the National Suicide Prevention Lifeline number in your phone so it's there when you need it: 1-800-273-TALK (8255). You can also help make a connection with a trusted individual like a family member, friend, spiritual advisor, or

mental health professional.

5. **Stay Connected:** Staying in touch after a crisis or after being discharged from care can make a difference. Studies have shown the number of suicide deaths goes down when someone follows up with the at-risk person.

MORE IDEAS

Instant access: It may be helpful to save several emergency numbers to your cell phone. The ability to get immediate help for yourself or for a friend can make a difference. The phone number for a trusted friend or relative

- The non-emergency number for the local police department
- The Crisis Text Line: 741741
- The National Suicide Prevention Lifeline: 1-800-273-TALK (8255).

Social Media: Knowing how to get help for a social media friend can save a life. Contact the social media site directly if you are concerned about a friend's updates or dial 911 in an emergency.

Treatments and Therapies

Research has shown that there are multiple risk factors for suicide and that these factors may vary with age, gender, physical and mental well-being, and with individual experiences. Treatments and therapies for people with suicidal thoughts or actions will vary as well.

Psychotherapies

Multiple types of psychosocial interventions have been found to be beneficial for individuals who have attempted suicide. These types of interventions may prevent someone from making another attempt. Psychotherapy, or "talk therapy," is one type of psychosocial intervention and can effectively reduce suicide risk.

One type of psychotherapy is called cognitive behavioral therapy (CBT). CBT can help people learn new ways of dealing with stressful experiences through training. CBT helps individuals recognize their own thought patterns and consider alternative actions when thoughts of suicide arise

Another type of psychotherapy, called dialectical behavior therapy (DBT), has been shown to reduce the rate of suicide among people with borderline personality disorder, a serious mental illness characterized by unstable moods, relationships, self-image, and behavior. A therapist trained in DBT helps a person recognize when his or her feelings or actions are disruptive or unhealthy, and teaches the skills needed to deal better with upsetting situations.

Medication

Some individuals at risk for suicide might benefit from medication. Doctors and patients can work together to find the best medication or medication combination, as well as the right dose.

Clozapine, is an antipsychotic medication used primarily to treat individuals with schizophrenia. However, it is the only medication with a specific U.S. Food and Drug Administration (FDA) indication for reducing the risk of recurrent suicidal behavior in patients with schizophrenia or schizoaffective disorder who are at risk for ongoing suicidal behavior. Because many individuals at risk for suicide often have psychiatric and substance use problems, individuals might benefit from medication along with psychosocial intervention.

If you are prescribed a medication, be sure you:

- Talk with your doctor or a pharmacist to make sure you understand the risks and benefits of the medications you're taking.

- Do not stop taking a medication without talking to your doctor first. Suddenly stopping a medication may lead to "rebound" or worsening of symptoms. Other uncomfortable or potentially dangerous withdrawal effects also are possible.

- Report any concerns about side effects to your doctor right away. You may need a change in the dose or a different medication.

- Report serious side effects to the U.S. Food and Drug Administration (FDA) MedWatch Adverse Event

Reporting program online or by phone at 1-800-332-1088. You or your doctor may send a report.

Other medications have been used to treat suicidal thoughts and behaviors but more research is needed to show the benefit for these options.

Ongoing Research

In order to know who is most at risk and to prevent suicide, scientists need to understand the role of long-term factors (such as childhood experiences) as well as more immediate factors like mental health and recent life events. Researchers also are looking at how genes can either increase risk or make someone more resilient to loss and hardships.

IF YOU KNOW SOMEONE IN CRISIS

Call the toll-free National Suicide Prevention Lifeline

(NSPL) at 1-800-273-TALK (8255), 24 hours a day, 7 days a week. The service is available to everyone. The deaf and hard of hearing can contact the Lifeline via TTY at 1-800-799-4889. All calls are confidential. Contact social media outlets directly if you are concerned about a friend's social media updates or dial 911 in an emergency. Learn more on the NSPL's website.

5

DEPRESSION

Depression (major depressive disorder or clinical depression) is a common but serious mood disorder. It causes severe symptoms that affect how you feel, think, and handle daily activities, such as sleeping, eating, or working. To be diagnosed with depression, the symptoms must be present for at least two weeks.

Some forms of depression are slightly different, or they may develop under unique circumstances, such as:

- Persistent depressive disorder (also called dysthymia) is a depressed mood that lasts for at least two years. A person diagnosed with persistent depressive disorder may have episodes of major depression along with periods of less severe symptoms, but symptoms must last for two years to be considered persistent depressive disorder.
- Postpartum depression is much more serious than the "baby blues" (relatively mild depressive and anxiety symptoms that typically clear within two weeks after

delivery) that many women experience after giving birth. Women with postpartum depression experience full-blown major depression during pregnancy or after delivery (postpartum depression). The feelings of extreme sadness, anxiety, and exhaustion that accompany postpartum depression may make it difficult for these new mothers to complete daily care activities for themselves and/or for their babies.

- Psychotic depression occurs when a person has severe depression plus some form of psychosis, such as having disturbing false fixed beliefs (delusions) or hearing or seeing upsetting things that others cannot hear or see (hallucinations). The psychotic symptoms typically have a depressive "theme," such as delusions of guilt, poverty, or illness.

- Seasonal affective disorder is characterized by the onset of depression during the winter months, when there is less natural sunlight. This depression generally lifts during spring and summer. Winter depression, typically accompanied by social withdrawal, increased sleep, and weight gain, predictably returns every year in seasonal affective disorder.

- Bipolar disorder is different from depression, but it is included in this list is because someone with bipolar disorder experiences episodes of extremely low moods that meet the criteria for major depression (called "bipolar depression"). But a person with bipolar disorder also experiences extreme high – euphoric or irritable – moods called "mania" or a less severe form called "hypomania."

Examples of other types of depressive disorders newly added to the diagnostic classification of DSM-5 include disruptive mood dys regulation disorder (diagnosed in children and adolescents) and premenstrual dysphoric disorder (PMDD).

Signs and Symptoms

If you have been experiencing some of the following signs and symptoms most of the day, nearly every day, for at least two weeks, you may be suffering from depression:

- Persistent sad, anxious, or "empty" mood
- Feelings of hopelessness, or pessimism
- Irritability
- Feelings of guilt, worthlessness, or helplessness
- Loss of interest or pleasure in hobbies and activities
- Decreased energy or fatigue
- Moving or talking more slowly
- Feeling restless or having trouble sitting still
- Difficulty concentrating, remembering, or making decisions
- Difficulty sleeping, early-morning awakening, or oversleeping
- Appetite and/or weight changes
- Thoughts of death or suicide, or suicide attempts
- Aches or pains, headaches, cramps, or digestive

problems without a clear physical cause and/or that do not ease even with treatment

Not everyone who is depressed experiences every symptom. Some people experience only a few symptoms while others may experience many. Several persistent symptoms in addition to low mood are required for a diagnosis of major depression, but people with only a few – but distressing – symptoms may benefit from treatment of their "subsyndromal" depression. The severity and frequency of symptoms and how long they last will vary depending on the individual and his or her particular illness. Symptoms may also vary depending on the stage of the illness.

Risk Factors

Depression is one of the most common mental disorders in the U.S. Current research suggests that depression is caused by a combination of genetic, biological, environmental, and psychological factors.

Depression can happen at any age, but often begins in

adulthood. Depression is now recognized as occurring in children and adolescents, although it sometimes presents with more prominent irritability than low mood. Many chronic mood and anxiety disorders in adults begin as high levels of anxiety in children.

Depression, especially in midlife or older adults, can co-occur with other serious medical illnesses, such as diabetes, cancer, heart disease, and Parkinson's disease. These conditions are often worse when depression is present. Sometimes medications taken for these physical illnesses may cause side effects that contribute to depression. A doctor experienced in treating these complicated illnesses can help work out the best treatment strategy.

Risk Factors Include:

- Personal or family history of depression
- Major life changes, trauma, or stress
- Certain physical illnesses and medications

Treatment and Therapies

Depression, even the most severe cases, can be treated. The earlier that treatment can begin, the more effective it is. Depression is usually treated with medications, psychotherapy, or a combination of the two. If these treatments do not reduce symptoms, electroconvulsive therapy (ECT) and other brain stimulation therapies may be options to explore.

No two people are affected the same way by depression and there is no "one-size-fits-all" for treatment. It may take some trial and error to find the treatment that works best for you.

Medications

Antidepressants are medicines that treat depression. They may help improve the way your brain uses certain chemicals that control mood or stress. You may need to try several different antidepressant medicines before finding the one that improves your symptoms and has manageable side effects. A medication that has helped you or a close family member in the past will often be considered.

Antidepressants take time – usually 2 to 4 weeks – to work, and often, symptoms such as sleep, appetite, and concentration problems improve before mood lifts, so it is important to give medication a chance before reaching a conclusion about its effectiveness. If you begin taking antidepressants, do not stop taking them without the help of a doctor. Sometimes people taking antidepressants feel better and then stop taking the medication on their own, and the depression returns. When you and your doctor have decided it is time to stop the medication, usually after a course of 6 to 12 months, the doctor will help you slowly and safely decrease your dose. Stopping them abruptly can cause withdrawal symptoms.

PLEASE NOTE:

In some cases, children, teenagers, and young adults under 25 may experience an increase in suicidal thoughts or behavior when taking antidepressants, especially in the first few weeks after starting or when the dose is changed. This warning from the U.S. Food and Drug Administration (FDA) also says that patients of all ages taking antidepressants should be watched closely, especially during the first few weeks of treatment.

If you are considering taking an antidepressant and you are pregnant, planning to become pregnant, or breastfeeding, talk to your doctor about any increased health risks to you or your unborn or nursing child.

You may have heard about an herbal medicine called St. John's wort. Although it is a top-selling botanical product, the FDA has not approved its use as an over-the-counter or prescription medicine for depression, and there are serious concerns about its safety (it should never be combined with a prescription antidepressant) and effectiveness. Do not use St. John's wort before talking to your health care provider. Other natural products sold as dietary supplements, including omega-3 fatty acids and S-adenosylmethionine (SAMe), remain under study but have not yet been proven safe and effective for routine use.

PSYCHOTHERAPIES

Several types of psychotherapy (also called "talk therapy" or, in a less specific form, counseling) can help people with depression. Examples of evidence-based approaches specific to the treatment of depression include cognitive-behavioral therapy (CBT), interpersonal therapy (IPT), and problem-solving therapy.

Brain Stimulation Therapies

If medications do not reduce the symptoms of depression, electroconvulsive therapy (ECT) may be an option to explore. Based on the latest research:

- ECT can provide relief for people with severe depression who have not been able to feel better with other treatments.
- Electroconvulsive therapy can be an effective treatment for depression. In some severe cases where

a rapid response is necessary or medications cannot be used safely, ECT can even be a first-line intervention.

- Once strictly an inpatient procedure, today ECT is often performed on an outpatient basis. The treatment consists of a series of sessions, typically three times a week, for two to four weeks.

- ECT may cause some side effects, including confusion, disorientation, and memory loss. Usually these side effects are short-term, but sometimes memory problems can linger, especially for the months around the time of the treatment course. Advances in ECT devices and methods have made modern ECT safe and effective for the vast majority of patients. Talk to your doctor and make sure you understand the potential benefits and risks of the treatment before giving your informed consent to undergoing ECT.

- ECT is not painful, and you cannot feel the electrical impulses. Before ECT begins, a patient is put under brief anesthesia and given a muscle relaxant. Within one hour after the treatment session, which takes only a few minutes, the patient is awake and alert.

Other more recently introduced types of brain stimulation therapies used to treat medicine-resistant depression include repetitive transcranial magnetic stimulation (rTMS) and vagus nerve stimulation (VNS). Other types of brain stimulation treatments are under study.

If you think you may have depression, start by making an appointment to see your doctor or health care provider. This could be your primary care practitioner or a health provider who specializes in diagnosing and treating mental health conditions.

Beyond Treatment: Things You Can Do

Here are other tips that may help you or a loved one during treatment for depression:

- Try to be active and exercise.
- Set realistic goals for yourself.

- Try to spend time with other people and confide in a trusted friend or relative.
- Try not to isolate yourself, and let others help you.
- Expect your mood to improve gradually, not immediately.
- Postpone important decisions, such as getting married or divorced, or changing jobs until you feel better. Discuss decisions with others who know you well and have a more objective view of your situation.
- Continue to educate yourself about depression.

JOIN A STUDY

What are Clinical Trials?

Clinical trials are research studies that look at new ways to prevent, detect, or treat diseases and conditions, including depression. During clinical trials, some participants receive treatments under study that might be new drugs or new combinations of drugs, new surgical procedures or devices, or new ways to use existing treatments. Other participants (in the "control group") receive a standard treatment, such as a medication already on the market, an inactive placebo medication, or no treatment. The goal of clinical trials is to determine if a new test or treatment works and is safe. Although individual participants may benefit from being part of a clinical trial, participants should be aware that the primary purpose of a clinical trial is to gain new scientific knowledge so that others may be better helped in the future.

PLEASE NOTE:

Decisions about whether to participate in a clinical trial, and which ones are best suited for a given individual, are best made in collaboration with your licensed health professional.

How Do I Find a Clinical Trial Near Me?

To search for a clinical trial near you, you can visit ClinicalTrials.gov. This is a searchable registry and results database of federally and privately supported clinical trials conducted in the United States and around the world (search:

depression). ClinicalTrials.gov gives you information about a trial's purpose, who may participate, locations, and contact information for more details. This information should be used in conjunction with advice from health professionals.

6
Attention Deficit Hyperactivity Disorder

Attention-deficit/hyperactivity disorder (ADHD) is a brain

disorder marked by an ongoing pattern of inattention and/or hyperactivity-impulsivity that interferes with functioning or development.

- Inattention means a person wanders off task, lacks persistence, has difficulty sustaining focus, and is disorganized; and these problems are not due to defiance or lack of comprehension.
- Hyperactivity means a person seems to move about constantly, including in situations in which it is not appropriate; or excessively fidgets, taps, or talks. In adults, it may be extreme restlessness or wearing others out with constant activity.
- Impulsivity means a person makes hasty actions that occur in the moment without first thinking about them and that may have high potential for harm; or a desire for immediate rewards or inability to delay gratification. An impulsive person may be socially intrusive and excessively interrupt others or make important decisions without considering the long-term consequences.

Signs and Symptoms

Inattention and hyperactivity/impulsivity are the key behaviors of ADHD. Some people with ADHD only have problems with one of the behaviors, while others have both inattention and hyperactivity-impulsivity. Most children have the combined type of ADHD.

In preschool, the most common ADHD symptom is hyperactivity.

It is normal to have some inattention, unfocused motor activity and impulsivity, but for people with ADHD, these behaviors:

- are more severe
- occur more often
- interfere with or reduce the quality of how they functions socially, at school, or in a job

Inattention

People with symptoms of inattention may often:

- Overlook or miss details, make careless mistakes in schoolwork, at work, or during other activities
- Have problems sustaining attention in tasks or play, including conversations, lectures, or lengthy reading
- Not seem to listen when spoken to directly
- Not follow through on instructions and fail to finish schoolwork, chores, or duties in the workplace or start tasks but quickly lose focus and get easily sidetracked
- Have problems organizing tasks and activities, such as what to do in sequence, keeping materials and belongings in order, having messy work and poor time management, and failing to meet deadlines
- Avoid or dislike tasks that require sustained mental effort, such as schoolwork or homework, or for teens and older adults, preparing reports, completing forms or reviewing lengthy papers
- Lose things necessary for tasks or activities, such as school supplies, pencils, books, tools, wallets, keys,

paperwork, eyeglasses, and cell phones
- Be easily distracted by unrelated thoughts or stimuli
- Be forgetful in daily activities, such as chores, errands, returning calls, and keeping appointments

Hyperactivity-Impulsivity

People with symptoms of hyperactivity-impulsivity may often:

- Fidget and squirm in their seats
- Leave their seats in situations when staying seated is expected, such as in the classroom or in the office
- Run or dash around or climb in situations where it is inappropriate or, in teens and adults, often feel restless
- Be unable to play or engage in hobbies quietly
- Be constantly in motion or "on the go," or act as if "driven by a motor"
- Talk nonstop
- Blurt out an answer before a question has been completed, finish other people's sentences, or speak without waiting for a turn in conversation

- Have trouble waiting his or her turn
- Interrupt or intrude on others, for example in conversations, games, or activities

Diagnosis of **ADHD** requires a comprehensive evaluation by a licensed clinician, such as a pediatrician, psychologist, or psychiatrist with expertise in **ADHD**. For a person to receive a diagnosis of **ADHD,** the symptoms of inattention and/or hyperactivity-impulsivity must be chronic or long-lasting, impair the person's functioning, and cause the person to fall behind normal development for his or her age. The doctor will also ensure that any **ADHD** symptoms are not due to another medical or psychiatric condition. Most children with **ADHD** receive a diagnosis during the elementary school years. For an adolescent or adult to receive a diagnosis of **ADHD**, the symptoms need to have been present prior to age 12.

ADHD symptoms can appear as early as between the ages of 3 and 6 and can continue through adolescence and adulthood. Symptoms of **ADHD** can be mistaken for emotional or disciplinary problems or missed entirely in quiet, well-behaved children, leading to a delay in diagnosis. Adults with undiagnosed **ADHD** may have a history of poor academic performance, problems at work, or difficult or failed relationships.

ADHD symptoms can change over time as a person ages. In young children with **ADHD**, hyperactivity-impulsivity is the most predominant symptom. As a child reaches elementary school, the symptom of inattention may become more prominent and cause the child to struggle academically. In adolescence, hyperactivity seems to lessen and may show more often as feelings of restlessness or fidgeting, but inattention and impulsivity may remain. Many adolescents with **ADHD** also struggle with relationships and antisocial behaviors. Inattention, restlessness, and impulsivity tend to persist into adulthood.

RISK FACTORS

Scientists are not sure what causes ADHD. Like many other

illnesses, a number of factors can contribute to ADHD, such as:

- Genes
- Cigarette smoking, alcohol use, or drug use during pregnancy
- Exposure to environmental toxins during pregnancy
- Exposure to environmental toxins, such as high levels of lead, at a young age
- Low birth weight
- Brain injuries

ADHD is more common in males than females, and females with **ADHD** are more likely to have problems primarily with inattention. Other conditions, such as learning disabilities, anxiety disorder, conduct disorder, depression, and substance abuse, are common in people with **ADHD.**

Treatment and Therapies

While there is no cure for ADHD, currently available treatments can help reduce symptoms and improve functioning. Treatments include medication, psychotherapy, education or training, or a combination of treatments.

Medication

For many people, ADHD medications reduce hyperactivity and impulsivity and improve their ability to focus, work, and learn. Medication also may improve physical coordination. Sometimes several different medications or dosages must be tried before finding the right one that works for a particular person. Anyone taking medications must be monitored closely and carefully by their prescribing doctor.

Stimulants. The most common type of medication used for treating ADHD is called a "stimulant." Although it may seem unusual to treat ADHD with a medication that is considered a stimulant, it works because it increases the brain chemicals dopamine and norepinephrine, which play essential roles in thinking and attention.

Under medical supervision, stimulant medications are considered safe. However, there are risks and side effects, especially when misused or taken in excess of the prescribed dose. For example, stimulants can raise blood pressure and heart rate and increase anxiety. Therefore, a person with other health problems, including high blood pressure, seizures, heart disease, glaucoma, liver or kidney disease, or an anxiety disorder should tell their doctor before taking a stimulant.

Talk with a doctor if you see any of these side effects while taking stimulants:

- decreased appetite
- sleep problems
- tics (sudden, repetitive movements or sounds);
- personality changes
- increased anxiety and irritability
- stomachaches
- headaches

NON-STIMULANTS

A few other ADHD medications are non-stimulants. These

medications take longer to start working than stimulants, but can also improve focus, attention, and impulsivity in a person with ADHD. Doctors may prescribe a non-stimulant: when a person has bothersome side effects from stimulants; when a stimulant was not effective; or in combination with a stimulant to increase effectiveness.

Although not approved by the U.S. Food and Drug Administration (FDA) specifically for the treatment of ADHD, some antidepressants are sometimes used alone or in combination with a stimulant to treat ADHD. Antidepressants may help all of the symptoms of ADHD and can be prescribed if a patient has bothersome side effects from stimulants. Antidepressants can be helpful in combination with stimulants if a patient also has another condition, such as an anxiety disorder, depression, or another mood disorder.

Doctors and patients can work together to find the best medication, dose, or medication combination.

Psychotherapy

Adding psychotherapy to treat ADHD can help patients and their families to better cope with everyday problems.

Behavioral therapy is a type of psychotherapy that aims to help a person change his or her behavior. It might involve practical assistance, such as help organizing tasks or completing schoolwork, or working through emotionally difficult events. Behavioral therapy also teaches a person how to:

- monitor his or her own behavior
- give oneself praise or rewards for acting in a desired way, such as controlling anger or thinking before acting

Parents, teachers, and family members also can give positive or negative feedback for certain behaviors and help establish clear rules, chore lists, and other structured routines to help a person control his or her behavior. Therapists may also teach children social skills, such as how to wait their turn, share toys, ask for help, or respond to teasing. Learning to read facial expressions and the tone of voice in others, and how to respond appropriately can also be part of social skills training.

Cognitive behavioral therapy can also teach a person mindfulness techniques, or meditation. A person learns how to be aware and accepting of one's own thoughts and feelings to improve focus and concentration. The therapist also encourages the person with ADHD to adjust to the life changes that come with treatment, such as thinking before acting, or resisting the urge to take unnecessary risks.

Family and marital therapy can help family members and spouses find better ways to handle disruptive behaviors, to encourage behavior changes, and improve interactions with the patient.

Education and Training

Children and adults with ADHD need guidance and understanding from their parents, families, and teachers to reach their full potential and to succeed. For school-age children, frustration, blame, and anger may have built up within a family before a child is diagnosed. Parents and children may need special help to overcome negative feelings. Mental health professionals can educate parents about ADHD and how it affects a family. They also will help the child and his or her parents develop new skills, attitudes, and ways of relating to each other.

Parenting skills training (behavioral parent management training) teaches parents the skills they need to encourage and reward positive behaviors in their children. It helps parents learn how to use a system of rewards and consequences to change a child's behavior. Parents are taught to give immediate and positive feedback for behaviors they want to encourage, and ignore or redirect behaviors that they want to discourage. They may also learn to structure situations in ways that support desired behavior.

Stress management techniques can benefit parents of children with ADHD by increasing their ability to deal with frustration so that they can respond calmly to their child's behavior.

Support groups can help parents and families connect with others who have similar problems and concerns. Groups often meet regularly to share frustrations and successes, to exchange information about recommended specialists and strategies, and to talk with experts.

Tips to Help Kids and Adults with ADHD Stay Organized

For Kids:

Parents and teachers can help kids with ADHD stay organized and follow directions with tools such as:

- Keeping a routine and a schedule. Keep the same routine every day, from wake-up time to bedtime. Include times for homework, outdoor play, and indoor activities. Keep the schedule on the refrigerator or on a bulletin board in the kitchen. Write changes on the schedule as far in advance as possible.

- Organizing everyday items. Have a place for everything, and keep everything in its place. This includes clothing, backpacks, and toys.
- Using homework and notebook organizers. Use organizers for school material and supplies. Stress to your child the importance of writing down assignments and bringing home the necessary books.
- Being clear and consistent. Children with ADHD need consistent rules they can understand and follow.
- Giving praise or rewards when rules are followed. Children with ADHD often receive and expect criticism. Look for good behavior, and praise it.

For Adults:

A professional counselor or therapist can help an adult with ADHD learn how to organize his or her life with tools such as:

- Keeping routines
- Making lists for different tasks and activities

- Using a calendar for scheduling events
- Using reminder notes
- Assigning a special place for keys, bills, and paperwork
- Breaking down large tasks into more manageable, smaller steps so that completing each part of the task provides a sense of accomplishment.

What is drug addiction?

Drug addiction is a chronic disease characterized by compulsive, or uncontrollable, drug seeking and use despite harmful consequences and changes in the brain, which can be long lasting. These changes in the brain can lead to the harmful behaviors seen in people who use drugs. Drug addiction is also a relapsing disease. Relapse is the return to drug use after an attempt to stop.

The path to drug addiction begins with the voluntary act of taking drugs. But over time, a person's ability to choose not to do so becomes compromised. Seeking and taking the drug becomes compulsive. This is mostly due to the effects of long-term drug exposure on brain function. Addiction affects parts of the brain involved in reward and motivation, learning and memory, and control over behavior. Addiction is a disease that affects both the brain and behavior.

Can drug addiction be treated?

Yes, but it's not simple. Because addiction is a chronic disease, people can't simply stop using drugs for a few days and be cured. Most patients need long-term or repeated care to stop using completely and recover their lives.

Addiction treatment must help the person do the following:

- stop using drugs
- stay drug-free
- be productive in the family, at work, and in society

Principles of Effective Treatment

Based on scientific research since the mid-1970s, the following key principles should form the basis of any effective treatment program:

- Addiction is a complex but treatable disease that affects brain function and behavior.

- No single treatment is right for everyone.
- People need to have quick access to treatment.
- Effective treatment addresses all of the patient's needs, not just his or her drug use.
- Staying in treatment long enough is critical.
- Counseling and other behavioral therapies are the most commonly used forms of treatment.
- Medications are often an important part of treatment, especially when combined with behavioral therapies.
- Treatment plans must be reviewed often and modified to fit the patient's changing needs.
- Treatment should address other possible mental disorders.
- Medically assisted detoxification is only the first stage of treatment.
- Treatment doesn't need to be voluntary to be effective.
- Drug use during treatment must be monitored continuously.
- Treatment programs should test patients for HIV/AIDS, hepatitis B and C, tuberculosis, and other

infectious diseases as well as teach them about steps they can take to reduce their risk of these illnesses.

What Are Treatments For Drug Addiction?

There are many options that have been successful in treating drug addiction, including:

- behavioral counseling
- medication
- medical devices and applications used to treat withdrawal symptoms or deliver skills training
- evaluation and treatment for co-occurring mental health issues such as depression and anxiety
- long-term follow-up to prevent relapse

A range of care with a tailored treatment program and follow-up options can be crucial to success. Treatment should include both medical and mental health services as needed. Follow-up care may include community- or family-based recovery support systems.

How are medications and devices used in drug addiction treatment?

Medications and devices can be used to manage withdrawal symptoms, prevent relapse, and treat co-occurring conditions.

Withdrawal. Medications and devices can help suppress withdrawal symptoms during detoxification. Detoxification is not in itself "treatment," but only the first step in the process. Patients who do not receive any further treatment after detoxification usually resume their drug use. One study of treatment facilities found that medications were used in almost 80 percent of detoxifications. In November 2017, the FDA granted a new indication to an electronic stimulation device, NSS-2 Bridge, for use in helping reduce opioid withdrawal symptoms. This device is placed behind the ear and sends electrical impulses to stimulate certain brain nerves.

Relapse Prevention:

Patients can use medications to help re-establish normal brain function and decrease cravings. Medications are available for treatment of opioid (heroin, prescription pain relievers), tobacco (nicotine), and alcohol addiction. Scientists are developing other medications to treat stimulant (cocaine, methamphetamine) and cannabis (marijuana) addiction. People who use more than one drug, which is very common, need treatment for all of the substances they use.

- *Opioids:* Methadone (Dolophine®, Methadose®), buprenorphine (Suboxone®, Subutex®, Probuphine® , Sublocade™), and naltrexone (Vivitrol®) are used to treat opioid addiction. Acting on the same targets in the brain as heroin and morphine, methadone and buprenorphine suppress withdrawal symptoms and
- relieve cravings. Naltrexone blocks the effects of opioids at their receptor sites in the brain and should be used only in patients who have already been

detoxified. All medications help patients reduce drug seeking and related criminal behavior and help them become more open to behavioral treatments. A NIDA study found that once treatment is initiated, both a buprenorphine/naloxone combination and an extended release naltrexone formulation are similarly effective in treating opioid addiction. Because full detoxification is necessary for treatment with naloxone, initiating treatment among active users was difficult, but once detoxification was complete, both medications had similar effectiveness.

- *Tobacco:* Nicotine replacement therapies have several forms, including the patch, spray, gum, and lozenges. These products are available over the counter. The U.S. FDA has approved two prescription medications for nicotine addiction: bupropion (Zyban®) and varenicline (Chantix®). They work differently in the brain, but both help prevent relapse in people trying to quit. The medications are more effective when combined with behavioral treatments, such as group and individual therapy as well as telephone quit lines.

ALCOHOL

Three medications have been FDA-approved for treating alcohol addiction and a fourth, topiramate, has shown promise in clinical trials (large-scale studies with people). The three approved medications are as follows:

- Naltrexone blocks opioid receptors that are involved in the rewarding effects of drinking and in the craving for alcohol. It reduces relapse to heavy drinking and is highly effective in some patients. Genetic differences may affect how well the drug works in certain patients.
- Acamprosate (Campral®) may reduce symptoms of long-lasting withdrawal, such as insomnia, anxiety, restlessness, and dysphoria (generally feeling unwell or unhappy). It may be more effective in patients with

severe addiction.

- Disulfiram (Antabuse®) interferes with the breakdown of alcohol. Acetaldehyde builds up in the body, leading to unpleasant reactions that include flushing (warmth and redness in the face), nausea, and irregular heartbeat if the patient drinks alcohol. Compliance (taking the drug as prescribed) can be a problem, but it may help patients who are highly motivated to quit drinking.
- *Co-occuring conditions:* Other medications are available to treat possible mental health conditions, such as depression or anxiety, that may be contributing to the person's addiction.

How are behavioral therapies used to treat drug addiction?

Behavioral therapies help patients:

- modify their attitudes and behaviors related to drug

use
- increase healthy life skills
- persist with other forms of treatment, such as medication

Patients can receive treatment in many different settings with various approaches.

Outpatient behavioral treatment includes a wide variety of programs for patients who visit a behavioral health counselor on a regular schedule. Most of the programs involve individual or group drug counseling, or both. These programs typically offer forms of behavioral therapy such as:

- **cognitive-behavioral therapy,** which helps patients recognize, avoid, and cope with the situations in which they are most likely to use drugs
- **multidimensional family therapy**—developed for adolescents with drug abuse problems as well as their families—which addresses a range of influences on

their drug abuse patterns and is designed to improve overall family functioning
- **Motivational Interviewing**, which makes the most of people's readiness to change their behavior and enter treatment
- **Motivational Incentives** (contingency management), which uses positive reinforcement to encourage abstinence from drugs

Treatment is sometimes intensive at first, where patients attend multiple outpatient sessions each week. After completing intensive treatment, patients transition to regular outpatient treatment, which meets less often and for fewer hours per week to help sustain their recovery. In September 2017, the FDA permitted marketing of the first mobile application, reSET®, to help treat substance use disorders. This application is intended to be used with outpatient treatment to treat alcohol, cocaine, marijuana, and stimulant substance use disorders. In September 2017, the FDA permitted marketing of the first mobile application, reSET®, to help treat substance use disorders.

This application is intended to be used with outpatient treatment to treat alcohol, cocaine, marijuana, and stimulant substance use disorders.

Inpatient or residential treatment can also be very effective, especially for those with more severe problems (including co-occurring disorders). Licensed residential treatment facilities offer 24-hour structured and intensive care, including safe housing and medical attention. Residential treatment facilities may use a variety of therapeutic approaches, and they are generally aimed at helping the patient live a drug-free, crime-free lifestyle after treatment. Examples of residential treatment settings include:

- **Therapeutic Communities**, which are highly structured programs in which patients remain at a residence, typically for 6 to 12 months. The entire community, including treatment staff and those in recovery, act as key agents of change, influencing the patient's attitudes, understanding, and behaviors associated with drug use.

- ***Shorter-term Residential Treatment,*** which typically focuses on detoxification as well as providing initial intensive counseling and preparation for treatment in a community-based setting.

- **Recovery Housing**, which provides supervised, short-term housing for patients, often following other types of inpatient or residential treatment. Recovery housing can help people make the transition to an independent life—for example, helping them learn how to manage finances or seek employment, as well as connecting them to support services in the community.

Is treatment different for criminal justice populations?

Scientific research since the mid-1970s shows that drug abuse treatment can help many drug-using offenders change their attitudes, beliefs, and behaviors towards drug abuse; avoid relapse; and successfully remove themselves from a life of substance abuse and crime. Many of the principles of treating drug addiction are similar for people within the criminal justice system as for those in the general population. However, many offenders don't have access to the types of services they need. Treatment that is of poor quality or is not well suited to the needs of offenders may not be effective at reducing drug use and criminal behavior.

In addition to the general principles of treatment, some considerations specific to offenders include the following:

- Treatment should include development of specific cognitive skills to help the offender adjust attitudes and beliefs that lead to drug abuse and crime, such as feeling entitled to have things one's own way or not understanding the consequences of one's behavior. This includes skills related to thinking, understanding, learning, and remembering.

- Treatment planning should include tailored services within the correctional facility as well as transition to community-based treatment after release.
- Ongoing coordination between treatment providers and courts or parole and probation officers is important in addressing the complex needs of offenders reentering society.

Challenges of Re-Entry

Drug abuse changes the function of the brain, and many things can "trigger" drug cravings within the brain. It's critical for those in treatment, especially those treated at an inpatient facility or prison, to learn how to recognize, avoid, and cope with triggers they are likely to be exposed to after treatment.

How many people get treatment for drug addiction?

According to SAMHSA's National Survey on Drug Use and Health, 22.5 million people (8.5 percent of the U.S. population) aged 12 or older needed treatment for an illicit drug or alcohol use problem in 2014. Only 4.2 million (18.5 percent of those who needed treatment) received any substance use treatment in the same year. Of these, about 2.6 million people received treatment at specialty treatment programs. The term "illicit" refers to the use of illegal drugs, including marijuana according to federal law, and misuse of prescription medications.

Points to Remember

- **Drug addiction can be treated, but it's not simple. Addiction treatment must help the person do the following:**
    - stop using drugs
    - stay drug-free
    - be productive in the family, at work, and in society

- **Successful treatment has several steps:**
    - detoxification
    - behavioral counseling
    - medication (for opioid, tobacco, or alcohol addiction)
    - evaluation and treatment for co-occurring mental health issues such as depression and anxiety
    - long-term follow-up to prevent relapse
- Medications and devices can be used to manage withdrawal symptoms, prevent relapse, and treat co-occurring conditions.
- **Behavioral therapies help patients:**
    - modify their attitudes and behaviors related to drug use
    - increase healthy life skills
    - persist with other forms of treatment, such as medication
- People within the criminal justice system may need additional treatment services to treat drug use

disorders effectively. However, many offenders don't have access to the types of services they need.

8

Obsessive-Compulsive Disorder

Obsessive-Compulsive Disorder: When Unwanted Thoughts or Irresistible Actions Take Over

Do you constantly have disturbing uncontrollable thoughts? Do you feel the urge to repeat the same behaviors or rituals over and over? Are these thoughts and behaviors making it hard for you to do things you enjoy?

If so, you may have obsessive-compulsive disorder (OCD). The good news is that, with treatment, you can overcome the fears and behaviors that may be putting your life on hold.

What is it like to have OCD?

"I couldn't do anything without my rituals. They invaded every aspect of my life. Counting really bogged me down. I would wash my hair three times because three was a good luck number for me. It took me longer to read because I'd have to count the lines in a paragraph. When I set my alarm at night, I had to set it to a time that wouldn't add up to a 'bad' number."

"Getting dressed in the morning was tough because I had to follow my routine or I would become very anxious and start getting dressed all over again." I always worried that if I didn't follow my routine, my parents were going to die. These thoughts triggered more anxiety and more rituals. Because of the time I spent on rituals, I was unable to do a lot of things that were important to me. I couldn't seem to overcome them until I got treatment."

What is OCD?

OCD is a common, chronic (long-lasting) disorder in which a person has uncontrollable, reoccurring thoughts (obsessions) and behaviors (compulsions) that he or she feels the urge to repeat over and over in response to the obsession.

While everyone sometimes feels the need to double check things, people with OCD have uncontrollable thoughts that cause them anxiety, urging them to check things repeatedly or perform routines and rituals for at least 1 hour per day. Performing the routines or rituals may bring brief but temporary relief from the anxiety. However, left untreated, these thoughts and rituals cause the person great distress and get in the way of work, school, and personal relationships.

What are the signs and symptoms of OCD?

People with OCD may have obsessions, compulsions, or both. Some people with OCD also have a tic disorder. Motor tics are sudden, brief, repetitive movements, such as eye blinking, facial grimacing, shoulder shrugging, or head or shoulder jerking. Common vocal tics include repetitive throat-clearing, sniffing, or grunting sounds.

Obsessions may include:

- Fear of germs or contamination

- Fear of losing or misplacing something

- Worries about harm coming towards oneself or others

- Unwanted and taboo thoughts involving sex, religion, or others

- Having things symmetrical or in perfect order

Compulsions May Include:

- Excessively cleaning or washing a body part

- Keeping or hoarding unnecessary objects

- Ordering or arranging items in a particular, precise

way

- Repeatedly checking on things, such as making sure that the door is locked or the oven is off
- Repeatedly counting items
- Constantly seeking reassurance

What causes OCD?

OCD may have a genetic component. It sometimes runs in families, but no one knows for sure why some family members have it while others don't. OCD usually begins in adolescence or young adulthood, and tends to appear at a younger age in boys than in girls. Researchers have found that several parts of the brain, as well as biological processes, play a key role in obsessive thoughts and compulsive behavior, as well as the fear and anxiety related to them. Researchers also know that people who have suffered physical or sexual trauma are at an increased risk for OCD.

Some children may develop a sudden onset or worsening of OCD symptoms after a streptococcal infection; this post-infectious autoimmune syndrome is called Pediatric Autoimmune **Neuropsychiatric Disorder Associated with Streptococcal Infections (PANDAS).**

How is OCD Treated?

The first step is to talk with your doctor or health care provider about your symptoms. The clinician should do an exam and ask you about your health history to make sure that a physical problem is not causing your symptoms. Your doctor may refer you to a mental health specialist, such as a psychiatrist, psychologist, social worker, or counselor for further evaluation or treatment.

OCD is generally treated with cognitive behavior therapy, medication, or both. Speak with your mental health professional about the best treatment for you.

Cognitive Behavioral Therapy (CBT)

In general, CBT teaches you different ways of thinking, behaving, and reacting to the obsessions and compulsions.

Exposure and Response Prevention (EX/RP) is a specific form of CBT which has been shown to help many patients recover from OCD. EX/RP involves gradually exposing you to your fears or obsessions and teaching you healthy ways to deal with the anxiety they cause.

Other therapies, such as habit reversal training, can also help you overcome compulsions.

For children, mental health professionals can also identify strategies to manage stress and increase support to avoid exacerbating OCD symptoms in school and home settings.

Medication

Doctors also may prescribe different types of medications to help treat OCD including selective serotonin reuptake inhibitors (SSRIs) and a type of serotonin reuptake inhibitor

(SRI) called clomipramine.

SSRIs and SRIs are commonly used to treat depression, but they are also helpful for the symptoms of OCD. SSRIs and SRIs may take 10 – 12 weeks to start working, longer than is required for the treatment of depression. These medications may also cause side effects, such as headaches, nausea, or difficulty sleeping.

People taking clomipramine, which is in a different class of medication from the SSRIs, sometimes experience dry mouth, constipation, rapid heartbeat, and dizziness on standing. These side effects are usually not severe for most people and improve as treatment continues, especially if the dose starts off low and is increased slowly over time. Talk to your doctor about any side effects that you have. Don't stop taking your medication without talking to your doctor first. Your doctor will work with you to find the best medication and dose for you.

Don't give up on treatment too quickly. Both psychotherapy and medication can take some time to work. While there is no cure for OCD, current treatments enable most people with this disorder to control their symptoms and lead full, productive lives. A healthy lifestyle that involves relaxation and managing stress can also help combat OCD. Make sure to also get enough sleep and exercise, eat a healthy diet, and turn to family and friends whom you trust for support.

9

Social Anxiety Disorder

Are you extremely afraid of being judged by others?

Are you very self-conscious in everyday social situations?

Do you avoid meeting new people?

If you have been feeling this way for at least six months and these feelings make it hard for you to do everyday tasks—such as talking to people at work or school—you may have a social anxiety disorder.

Social anxiety disorder (also called social phobia) is a mental health condition. It is an intense, persistent fear of being watched and judged by others. This fear can affect work, school, and your other day-to-day activities. It can even make it hard to make and keep friends. But social anxiety disorder doesn't have to stop you from reaching your potential. Treatment can help you overcome your symptoms.

What is it like having social anxiety disorder?

"In school, I was always afraid of being called on, even when I knew the answers. I didn't want people to think I was stupid or boring. My heart would pound and I would feel dizzy and sick. When I got a job, I hated to meet with my boss or talk in a meeting. I couldn't attend my best friend's wedding reception because I was afraid of having to meet new people. I tried to calm myself by drinking several glasses of wine before an event and then I started drinking every day to try to face what I had to do."

"I finally talked to my doctor because I was tired of feeling this way and I was worried that I would lose my job. I now take medicine and meet with a counselor to talk about ways to cope with my fears. I refuse to use alcohol to escape my fears and I'm on my way to feeling better."

What is social anxiety disorder?

Social anxiety disorder is a common type of anxiety disorder. A person with social anxiety disorder feels symptoms of anxiety or fear in certain or all social situations, such as meeting new people, dating, being on a job interview, answering a question in class, or having to talk to a cashier in a store. Doing everyday things in front of people—such as eating or drinking in front of others or using a public restroom—also causes anxiety or fear. The person is afraid that he or she will be humiliated, judged, and rejected.

The fear that people with social anxiety disorder have in social situations is so strong that they feel it is beyond their ability to control. As a result, it gets in the way of going to work, attending school, or doing everyday things. People with social anxiety disorder may worry about these and other things for weeks before they happen. Sometimes, they end up staying away from places or events where they think they might have to do something that will embarrass them.

Some people with the disorder do not have anxiety in social situations but have performance anxiety instead. They feel physical symptoms of anxiety in situations such as giving a speech, playing a sports game, or dancing or playing a musical instrument on stage.

Social anxiety disorder usually starts during youth in people who are extremely shy. Social anxiety disorder is not uncommon; research suggests that about 7 percent of Americans are affected. Without treatment, social anxiety disorder can last for many years or a lifetime and prevent a person from reaching his or her full potential.

What are the signs and symptoms of social anxiety disorder?

When having to perform in front of or be around others, people with social anxiety disorder tend to:

- Blush, sweat, tremble, feel a rapid heart rate, or feel their "mind going blank"
- Feel nauseous or sick to their stomach
- Show a rigid body posture, make little eye contact, or speak with an overly soft voice
- Find it scary and difficult to be with other people, especially those they don't already know, and have a hard time talking to them even though they wish they could
- Be very self-conscious in front of other people and feel embarrassed and awkward
- Be very afraid that other people will judge them
- Stay away from places where there are other people

What causes social anxiety disorder?

Social anxiety disorder sometimes runs in families, but no one knows for sure why some family members have it while others don't. Researchers have found that several parts of the brain are involved in fear and anxiety. Some researchers think that misreading of others' behavior may play a role in causing or worsening social anxiety. For example, you may think that people are staring or frowning at you when they truly are not. Underdeveloped social skills are another possible contributor to social anxiety. For example, if you have underdeveloped social skills, you may feel discouraged after talking with people and may worry about doing it in the future. By learning more about fear and anxiety in the brain, scientists may be able to create better treatments. Researchers are also looking for ways in which stress and environmental factors may play a role.

How is social anxiety disorder treated?

First, talk to your doctor or health care professional about your symptoms. Your doctor should do an exam and ask you about your health history to make sure that an unrelated physical problem is not causing your symptoms. Your doctor may refer you to a mental health specialist, such as a psychiatrist, psychologist, clinical social worker, or counselor. The first step to effective treatment is to have a diagnosis made, usually by a mental health specialist.

Social anxiety disorder is generally treated with psychotherapy (sometimes called "talk" therapy), medication, or both. Speak with your doctor or health care provider about the best treatment for you.

Psychotherapy

A type of psychotherapy called cognitive behavioral therapy (CBT) is especially useful for treating social anxiety disorder. CBT teaches you different ways of thinking, behaving, and reacting to situations that help you feel less anxious and fearful. It can also help you learn and practice social skills. CBT delivered in a group format can be especially helpful.

Support Groups

Many people with social anxiety also find support groups

helpful. In a group of people who all have social anxiety disorder, you can receive unbiased, honest feedback about how others in the group see you.

This way, you can learn that your thoughts about judgment and rejection are not true or are distorted. You can also learn how others with social anxiety disorder approach and overcome the fear of social situations.

Medication

There are three types of medications used to help treat social anxiety disorder:

- Anti-anxiety medications
- Antidepressants
- Beta-blockers

Anti-anxiety medications are powerful and begin working right away to reduce anxious feelings; however, these medications are usually not taken for long periods of time. People can build up a tolerance if they are taken over a long period of time and may need higher and higher doses to get the same effect. Some people may even become dependent on them. To avoid these problems, doctors usually prescribe anti-anxiety medications for short periods, a practice that is especially helpful for older adults.

Antidepressants are mainly used to treat depression, but are also helpful for the symptoms of social anxiety disorder. In contrast to anti-anxiety medications, they may take several weeks to start working. Antidepressants may also cause side effects, such as headaches, nausea, or difficulty sleeping. These side effects are usually not severe for most people, especially if the dose starts off low and is increased slowly over time. Talk to your doctor about any side effects that you have.

Beta-blockers are medicines that can help block some of the physical symptoms of anxiety on the body, such as an increased heart rate, sweating, or tremors. Beta-blockers are commonly the medications of choice for the "performance anxiety" type of social anxiety.

Your doctor will work with you to find the best medication,

dose, and duration of treatment. Many people with social anxiety disorder obtain the best results with a combination of medication and CBT or other psychotherapies.

Don't give up on treatment too quickly. Both psychotherapy and medication can take some time to work. A healthy lifestyle can also help combat anxiety. Make sure to get enough sleep and exercise, eat a healthy diet, and turn to family and friends who you trust for support.

10
EATING DISORDERS

Eating Disorders: About More Than Food

Has your urge to eat less or more food spiraled out of control?

Are you overly concerned about your outward appearance?

If so, you may have an eating disorder.

What are eating disorders?

Eating disorders are serious medical illnesses marked by severe disturbances to a person's eating behaviors.

Obsessions with food, body weight, and shape may be signs of an eating disorder. These disorders can affect a person's physical and mental health; in some cases, they can be life-threatening. But eating disorders can be treated. Learning more about them can help you spot the warning signs and seek treatment early.

Remember: Eating disorders are not a lifestyle choice. They are biologically-influenced medical illnesses.

Who is at risk for eating disorders?

Eating disorders can affect people of all ages, racial/ethnic backgrounds, body weights, and genders. Although eating disorders often appear during the teen years or young adulthood, they may also develop during childhood or later in life (40 years and older).

Remember: People with eating disorders may appear healthy, yet be extremely ill.

The exact cause of eating disorders is not fully understood, but research suggests a combination of genetic, biological, behavioral, psychological, and social factors can raise a person's risk.

What are the common types of eating disorders?

Common eating disorders include anorexia nervosa, bulimia nervosa, and binge-eating disorder. If you or someone you know experiences the symptoms listed below, it could be a sign of an eating disorder—call a health provider right away for help.

What is anorexia nervosa?

People with anorexia nervosa avoid food, severely restrict food, or eat very small quantities of only certain foods. Even when they are dangerously underweight, they may see themselves as overweight. They may also weigh themselves repeatedly.

There are two subtypes of anorexia nervosa: a *restrictive* subtype and *binge-purge* subtype.

Restrictive: People with the restrictive subtype of anorexia nervosa place severe restrictions on the amount and type of food they consume.

Binge-Purge: People with the binge-purge subtype of anorexia nervosa also place severe restrictions on the amount and type of food they consume. In addition, they may have binge eating and purging behaviors (such as vomiting, use of laxatives and diuretics, etc.).

Symptoms Include:

- Extremely restricted eating and/or intensive and excessive exercise
- Extreme thinness (emaciation)
- A relentless pursuit of thinness and unwillingness to maintain a normal or healthy weight
- Intense fear of gaining weight
- Distorted body image, a self-esteem that is heavily influenced by perceptions of body weight and shape, or a denial of the seriousness of low body weight

Over time, these symptoms may also develop:

- Thinning of the bones (osteopenia or osteoporosis)
- Mild anemia and muscle wasting and weakness
- Brittle hair and nails
- Dry and yellowish skin
- Growth of fine hair all over the body (lanugo)
- Severe constipation
- Low blood pressure, slowed breathing and pulse
- Damage to the structure and function of the heart
- Drop in internal body temperature, causing a person to feel cold all the time
- Lethargy, sluggishness, or feeling tired all the time
- Infertility
- Brain damage
- Multiorgan failure

Anorexia can be fatal. Anorexia nervosa has the highest mortality (death) rate of any mental disorder. People with anorexia may die from medical conditions and complications associated with starvation; by comparison, people with others eating disorders die of suicide. If you or someone you know is in crisis and needs immediate help, call the toll-free National Suicide Prevention Lifeline (NSPL) at 1-800-273-TALK (8255), 24 hours a day, 7 days a week.

What is bulimia nervosa?

People with bulimia nervosa have recurrent episodes of eating unusually large amounts of food and feeling a lack of control over these episodes. This binge-eating is followed by behaviors that compensate for the overeating, such as forced vomiting, excessive use of laxatives or diuretics, fasting, excessive exercise, or a combination of these behaviors. Unlike those with anorexia nervosa, people with bulimia nervosa may maintain a normal weight or be overweight.

Symptoms include:

- Chronically inflamed and sore throat
- Swollen salivary glands in the neck and jaw area
- Worn tooth enamel and increasingly sensitive and

decaying teeth (a result of exposure to stomach acid)
- Acid reflux disorder and other gastrointestinal problems
- Intestinal distress and irritation from laxative abuse
- Severe dehydration from purging
- Electrolyte imbalance (too low or too high levels of sodium, calcium, potassium and other minerals), which can lead to stroke or heart attack

What is binge-eating disorder?

People with binge-eating disorder lose control over their eating. Unlike bulimia nervosa, periods of binge-eating are not followed by purging, excessive exercise, or fasting. As a result, people with binge-eating disorder are often overweight or obese.

Symptoms Include:

- Eating unusually large amounts of food in a specific amount of time, such as a 2-hour period
- Eating fast during binge episodes

- Eating even when full or not hungry
- Eating until uncomfortably full
- Eating alone or in secret to avoid embarrassment
- Feeling distressed, ashamed, or guilty about eating
- Frequently dieting, possibly without weight loss

How are eating disorders treated?

It is important to seek treatment early for eating disorders. People with eating disorders are at higher risk for suicide and medical complications.

Some people with eating disorders may also have other mental disorders (such as depression or anxiety) or problems with substance use.

Treatment plans for eating disorders include psychotherapy, medical care and monitoring, nutritional counseling, medications, or a combination of these approaches. Typical treatment goals include restoring adequate nutrition, bringing weight to a healthy level, reducing excessive exercise, and stopping binge-purge and binge-eating behaviors. Complete recovery is possible.

Specific forms of psychotherapy (or "talk therapy") and cognitive behavioral approaches can be effective for treating specific eating disorders. For more about psychotherapies, visit www.nimh.nih.gov/health/topics/psychotherapies

Research also suggests that medications may help treat some eating disorders and co-occurring anxiety or depression related to eating disorders. Information about medications changes frequently, so talk to your health care professional at **The Raven Institute, Inc.** and check the U.S. Food and Drug Administration (FDA) website for the latest warnings, patient medication guides, or newly approved medications.

ABOUT THE AUTHOR

Troy Foskey Jr., PhD, NP, CAC, P.C. is the Founder & Director of: **The Raven Institute, Inc. - Raven Crisis-Care & Intervention,** a **Federally Registered 501c Non-Profit Corporation** located in Ludowici Georgia, US.

Dr. Troy Foskey Jr is a Veteran of both the United States Air Force & United States Army, serving as a Combat Medic, an MP, & an EMS Nurse, being honorably discharged in 2006 after 18 plus years of outstanding service. He was medically retired following service related injuries. He is a Health Psychologist, a Licensed Integrative Therapist, Certified Crisis Intervention Specialist, Natural Health

Practitioner, Certified Addiction Coach, Certified Holistic Life Coach, & an Ordained & Licensed Crisis Care Chaplain. as well as several other certifications in areas of Healthcare, Wellness & Psychology.

The 48 year old Medical Practitioner began his love of the medical profession while serving as a Combat medical Specialist in the US Military. He later completed his advanced nursing degree, specializing in emergency medicine and critical care.

Dr. Foskey has always held a keen interest & love of human psychology & Holistic Healthcare & Wellness, so after retiring from the US Military in 2006, he began working on his advanced training & education in Health Psychology, Crisis Intervention, Functional Medicine, & Holistic Wellness.

Dr. Foskey earned his Master's Degree in Naturopathic Medicine & Natural Health Science, his PhD in both Psychology & Theology, & he is currently working to complete his I-MD, Doctor of Integrative Medicine, which he will complete in August 2018.

The Raven Institute, Inc. specializes in several areas of Crisis Intervention, Mental Health Treatment, & Holistic Health & Wellness Services including, but not limited to, Life-Crisis Management/Intervention, Integrative Therapy, Addiction Management/Treatment Services, PTSD Management/Treatment, Holistic Health/Wellness Care & Consulting, Spiritual/Pastoral Counseling, Suicide Prevention, Marriage/Couples Counseling/Therapy, Family Counseling/Therapy, Animal Assisted Therapy, Anger Management/Counseling, Traumatic Event Therapy, & many other services including a variety of Life Coaching options, depending upon the wishes and/or assessments of the Patient/Client, such as Addiction Coaching, Wellness Coaching, & Holistic Life Coaching just to name a few. ***The Raven Institute, Inc.*** offers Secular & NonSecular Services (Non-Religion & Religion Based), depending upon the requests/needs of the Patient/Client.

The Raven Institute, Inc. is a proud member of several Professional Organizations & Certification Boards, including but not limited to, *The American Academy of Experts in Traumatic Stress, National Board of Medical Examiners (NBME), American Psychological Association (APA),*

International Association of Wellness Professionals (IAWP), The American Holistic Health Association (AHHA), The American Association of Drugless Practitioners (AADP), National Crisis Chaplains Association, National Association of Pastoral Counselors, & several other professional & speciality field related organizations.

Thank You to everyone who took the time to read my first Book:

The Unique Path: Life Crisis Management

I'm very grateful, & humbled by your support. I hope that you will find the information helpful, & please read my next book in the series due for release the first week of July 2018.

- **Dr. Troy Foskey Jr**

www.ingramcontent.com/pod-product-compliance
Lightning Source LLC
Chambersburg PA
CBHW020436220526
45464CB00002B/725